MASCULINIZING HORMONAL THERAPY FOR THE TRANSGENDERED

MASCULINIZING

HORMONAL THERAPY

FOR THE

TRANSGENDERED

Sheila Kirk, M.D.

Together Lifeworks
P.O. Box 38114
Blawnox, PA 15238-8114

Masculinizing Hormonal Therapy For The Transgendered

ISBN 1-887796-02-9

Published by:

Together Lifeworks®
P.O. Box 38114
Blawnox, PA 15238-8114

ABOUT THE AUTHOR

As a board certified obstetrician - gynecologist with over 25 years of medical experience in both private practice and research and as a transgendered person herself, Dr. Sheila Kirk is in a unique position to help the transgendered community improve their overall physical and emotional well-being while providing insight and instruction to the medical professionals who administer their care.

During her years in active practice in a major U.S. city, Dr. Kirk delivered over 8,000 babies; performed hundreds of related surgeries ranging from reconstructive gynecological concerns to infertility problems and became a leading expert in hormonal therapy for the pre-menopausal and post-menopausal biologic woman and the transgendered population.

Throughout her busy years as a sole practitioner, Dr. Kirk found time to share her knowledge and expertise with young medical students. For over twenty years, she served as Assistant Clinical Professor, lecturer and consultant at a major university medical school, teaching and supervising medical students and residents in obstetrics and gynecology. On several occasions throughout those years, she was recognized as Teacher of the Year by both the medical students and resident staff. She considers these awards amongst the highest honors she has received.

Dr. Kirk serves as the International Foundation for Gender Education's Director of the Division for Medical Liaison and Research instructing and advising members of both the transgendered and professional communities in the latest developments in transgendered care.

One of Dr. Kirk's primary interests is in generating and promoting research in a number of areas regarding the care of the transgendered person. Currently, Dr. Kirk is conducting two on-going research projects dealing with the teenage transgendered person and the post-operative transsexual. In addition, she is currently in the process of developing research in contragender hormonal therapy as it relates to lipid profiles and breast and prostate problems in the transgendered individual.

A noted author and lecturer, Dr. Kirk has written numerous books, articles and research reports on transgendered care as well as other medical concerns in her chosen discipline.

Sought after worldwide as a leading authority on transgendered issues, Dr. Kirk, lectures extensively at universities, medical conferences and related symposiums both nationally and internationally.

She is a member of the Harry Benjamin Association Gender Dysphoria Association, a member of the Board of Directors of the International Foundation of Gender Education and its Executive Committee, and serves on the editorial staff of AEGIS, an international transsexual support and resource foundation.

Dr. Kirk's web address is SheilaKirk@aol.com. You can write Dr. Kirk c/o Together Lifeworks, P.O. Box 38114, Blawnox, PA 15238-8114.

Other Publications by Sheila Kirk, M.D.:

Medical, Legal and Workplace Issues For Transsexuals,
co-authored by Martine Rothblatt, J.D.
©1995 Together Lifeworks®, Watertown, MA

Feminizing Hormonal Therapy For The Transgendered
©1996 Together Lifeworks®, Blawnox, PA

Hormones - Male to Female
©1994 edition Sheila Kirk, M.D.
(English/German/French/Spanish Translations)
International Foundation For Gender Education,
Waltham, MA

Hormones - Female to Male
©1994 edition Sheila Kirk, M.D.
(English/German/French/Spanish Translations)
International Foundation For Gender Education,
Waltham, MA

Hormonal Treatment For The Transsexual - An Overview For The Professional (audio cassette)
©1994 Sheila Kirk, M.D.
International Foundation For Gender Education,
Waltham, MA

Hormones - Male To Female, Female To Male
©1991, 1992 editions Sheila Kirk, M.D.
International Foundation For Gender Education,
Waltham, MA

How To Find A Physician
©1989 Sheila Kirk, M.D.
International Foundation For Gender Education,
Waltham, MA

How To Be A Good Medical Consumer
©1989 Sheila Kirk, M.D.
International Foundation For Gender Education,
Waltham, MA

TABLE OF CONTENTS

ACKNOWLEDGEMENTS

I'm exceedingly grateful to Pamela, my spouse, for her very knowledgeable review and contribution to the assembling of this book. Without her very capable and tireless attention, this book would not have come to print.

I wish to thank Lori, my office assistant for many years. I am very grateful for her generous assistance in the preparation of much of the basic material for this monograph. I want also to thank my very capable transcriptionist, Joan, for her tireless effort and patience with me in assembling this work.

INTRODUCTION

Through the years, a moderate amount of reporting has found its way into the various medical journals. In years past, the data was helpful to health-care professionals who care for the transgendered, but it was based on experience with small groups of individuals receiving therapy of various kinds. In modern times, medical reporting, while coming from a precious few researchers throughout the world, is much more meaningful, based on larger series of transgendered individuals who are observed for longer periods of time. This is what is important in developing therapy techniques, and it is very much the case with hormonal therapy of the transgendered female to male person.

The information compiled here for your review and education is presented in language selected for your more complete understanding and for your ability to be able to discuss all aspects of care with your physician. This information is based on medical research and reporting to the medical community. It is not taken from the transgendered literature which often carries with it myth, misinformation, and fantasy. With this in mind, what I am telling you is what is told to physicians by their colleagues when they read medical studies to educate themselves. They are accustomed to scientific language and detail. I will try very hard not to burden you with that kind of detail.

This book is for you truly—not your doctor. Your physician has access to the medical literature. Though I do understand how the medically trained can find this information a help in their care of you, the medical literature is available to them for more in-depth concept and information.

The data I give to you is meant to inform, not to frighten. I believe that most candidates for hormonal therapy can use a hormonal regimen with a high degree of safety, as long as they are evaluated adequately for hormonal use and then monitored on a regular basis so as to be certain that good health is maintained.

IT IS VERY IMPORTANT AS WELL THAT PATIENTS ON A HORMONAL REGIMEN ADHERE TO THE INSTRUCTIONS GIVEN THEM BY THEIR PHYSICIAN.

There are some precepts that must be emphasized at the very start, however, and they are meant to safeguard you, and to instill in you, a deep sense of reality as you follow this pathway to a contragender existence.

1. I want to give a very strict warning to those who would consider using hormonal medication prescribed for another person. This is not safe! ***Do not do it! Ever!***

2. A similar and even more forceful caution is given to those who would purchase their hormones from a black market source. Purchase of these medications from mail order houses that sell to anyone making inquiry is to be avoided. To purchase from sources in foreign countries and from vendors who claim that they can "get it for you", is a decided mistake. They are, in essence, pill pushers and very suspect in whatever they offer. The medication may not be pure. It may be contaminated. In essence, it could cause you great harm. Even more importantly, medication whether oral or injectable obtained this way, will cause one to bypass the important monitoring rendered by a qualified and knowledgeable medical

physician. This can only lead to very serious consequences. ***Don't do it!***

3. I urge you to take your prescriptions to a reputable pharmacy and to abide by the instructions given to you for their use. Don't double dose or alter the regimen without discussion with your doctor, for this can lead to serious problems. There should be room for discussion with your physician, and the medical expert with experience in transgendered medical care will know there are many ways to accomplish what is possible for you.

Individuals who do not follow these guidelines risk damaging their health. Granted, physicians who care and who are responsible and empathetic, are not always easy to find -- but they do exist. If you are tempted to take shortcuts or abbreviated pathways, please remember that good health is paramount and you must preserve it. Anything that risks good health is foolhardy and irrational.

The plan for this book is to give some insight into the subject of endocrinology, a branch of internal medicine that deals with special glands in our bodies which produce hormones. To be a little bit more thorough, we will describe briefly some of the anatomy and some of the biochemistry involved with production of the sex hormones, also known as sex steroids. Then there will be brief discussion of estrogen and its effect on the genetic female.

Next, we will discuss some of the physiology or function of the sex steroid, testosterone in the genetic male and show what it does for him. Following this, we will discuss how this hormone counteracts estrogen in the genetic female and reverses those changes brought about by estrogen production through the pubertal years. This, in fact, is the masculinization process.

Following this, we will discuss complications or problems encountered in hormonal use in the genetic female and then give insight into some of the hormonal regimens currently in use throughout the world. Chapters 4 and 8 deal with initial evaluation and follow-up or monitoring evaluations. They will indicate the importance of your adherence to periodic office and laboratory visits.

Important and frequently asked questions have been included and answered. These questions quite possibly could be ones you have wanted to ask and didn't know where to get accurate and honest answers.

Again my intent is simply to give you some basic knowledge so you can work more cooperatively with your physician and better understand his or her approach to you.

Chapter 1 A Little Anatomy and Biochemistry

To begin with, we ought to define the word hormone, since it is a such a special substance in the human body. Its involvement in human physiology is quite extensive, for it is a part of the growth and daily maintenance of the human body. Hormones are very much a part of reproduction. But hormones are necessary as well to our health and the quality of our lives.

A hormone is a complex chemical structure made in very minute amounts in specialized organs called glands. It is deposited directly into the bloodstream and is transported in a special manner to a target organ. There it exerts a very special and specific influence upon that target organ to function in a definite way. The target organ may be another hormone gland or other body tissue. The hormone enters that structure and influences it to function in a particular manner.

For instance, consider the male penis. It is a target organ that responds to the hormone testosterone as it is produced in the hormone gland, the testes. (The testes themselves are a target organ for the pituitary gland.) Under the influence of testosterone which is produced on a fairly regular basis, the penis as a reproductive organ changes in caliber and length during puberty. It will continue to be maintained by testicular production of testosterone in the years after puberty. For example, when there is appropriate visual or mental stimulus, testosterone will influence blood flow to be increased in the penis which will engorge it and cause erection. Testosterone will have influenced the testes to produce a very adequate supply of sperm and the fluid in which they are to be transferred. That fluid will come from the prostate and the seminal vesicles, accessory sex organs in the reproductive anatomy of the male. After penetration and with orgasm, an ejaculate is produced, which is composed of fluid and sperm. The sex act is then complete, all under the influence of testosterone.

But that is not all of the need for testosterone. Its production is vital in the maintenance and function of many other organs and tissues. The skin and the sebaceous glands, and sweat glands that are contained in the skin are target organs for testosterone. This hormone has direct effect on these structures along with many others inclusive of bone and muscle.

Special glands in our bodies make these hormones. They are included in the Endocrine System, and they are under the auspices of a master endocrine gland called the pituitary located very close to the brain. Even the pituitary is subject to another influence, a structure in the brain called the hypothalamus. The pituitary gland produces hormones that are called gonadotropins. They are specific to and stimulate other endocrine glands to act. They enter the bloodstream and are taken to the other endocrine glands by an elaborate transport system. The gonadotropins stimulate those glands to produce their own hormones, which in turn then exert effect upon target organs such as skin, bone, muscle, breast, reproductive tract structures, and a host of other tissues. The hormones influence target structures by way of a receptor system. Located on the surface of the many thousands of cells forming the target organ are receptors which either accept or reject the hormone presented. If accepted, the hormone enters each cell and causes reaction(s) that are characteristic for that target organ or tissue. It's very complicated but very efficient and exceedingly important to good health. As you will understand in the following, hormones enter into many body systems not just those having to do with being male or female.

The following is a list of the endocrine glands of the human body:

The Pituitary Gland

As mentioned earlier, the Pituitary Gland is under the control of a part of the brain known as the hypothalamus. It is in complex relationship with endocrine glands it influences to regulate the amounts of hormones that they produce. The pituitary gland is located on the undersurface of the brain and it makes a number of gonadotropin hormones:

Thyroid stimulating hormone.

Parathyroid stimulating hormone.

Adrenal stimulating hormones.

Ovarian stimulation hormones (follicle stimulating hormone, luteinizing hormone).

Testes stimulating hormones (follicle stimulating hormone, luteinizing hormone).

Growth hormone (most prominent at puberty).

The Thyroid Gland

This gland is located in the neck just beneath the male's "Adam's apple". The pituitary directs the thyroid to produce a hormone which influences metabolism and is responsible for growth of the body and maintenance of various tissues. It has a great deal to do with reproduction in the genetic female. Lack of adequate thyroid function leads to many changes in the way the gastrointestinal tract works. It also has control over the maintenance of the skin. Overactivity of the thyroid gland can lead to serious disease involving normal heart function.

The Parathyroid Glands

These glands, four in number, are located in the neck just in front of the thyroid gland. Their hormone production is involved with calcium and phosphorus metabolism, and therefore, they are vital to skeletal growth and continuing bone metabolism.

The Adrenal Glands

These glands are two in number and are located in the back on the very top of each kidney. Hormones from these glands are very involved with glucose (carbohydrate) metabolism and water and electrolyte balance. Electrolyte balance is vital to healthy cardiac function, to kidney and musculoskeletal activity and to various enzyme systems. They produce, in small amounts, the sex hormones, estrogen and testosterone in both males and females as well.

The Ovarian Glands

There are two ovaries located deep within the lower abdomen or pelvis of the female next to the uterus. The major hormones produced, estrogen and progesterone are not only part of the reproductive system, but are involved intimately in many other systems, for instance, bone and lipid metabolism, breast, skin, etc.

The Testicular Glands

The testes are located in a sac outside of the body called the scrotum, just beneath the penis. The major hormone, testosterone, produced in the testes is not only part of reproductive tract function, but very involved in many other organ systems; Bone metabolism, lipid profile and red blood cell production are only some of these. Certain cells in the testes produce testosterone and other specialized cells produce sperm cells. The pituitary has influence in several other systems which certainly can be considered as part of the endocrine system:

Prolactin - A hormone from the pituitary that takes part in the development of the female breast in puberty and which is very much the main influential factor in the production of breast milk during and after pregnancy. However, it is produced in males as well as females.

Pancreas - The pituitary gland is in balance with this organ in its production of insulin and with the adrenal gland in its hormonal influence upon glucose metabolism. If the balance is altered either a diabetic state or a blood sugar deficit state will develop (hypoglycemia).

Placenta - This organ though only a temporary one formed in a pregnancy is a virtual factory of hormone production. It assumes influence over the maintenance of the pregnancy replacing ovarian function after a certain period of time. This is over and above its primary activity in conducting nutrition and oxygen to the developing fetus.

At the risk of being too scientific, I'm going to show you the biochemical scheme for the production of **progesterone, testosterone**, and **estradiol** (estrogen) in the genetic female. Actually, this same scheme exists in both the genetic male and female. Because certain factors are involved, males produce much less estrogen and progesterone and females produce far less testosterone. Genetic influence determines prominence of one system over another. Note also that cholesterol is the precursor, or original chemical substance from which the hormones come. Our bodies can make two carbon segments (acetyl groups) and chemically join them together to form many different substances needed in our body including the hormones testosterone, estradiol (estrogen) and progesterone. Our bodies, however, prefer to use dietary cholesterol in various "breakdown" reactions to make the three hormones. **Cholesterol** is very important to us, for it takes part in some way in the metabolism or function of virtually all tissue in our bodies. The concern over it, has to do with its excess in our systems and the "pile up" in our arteries leading to vessel and heart disease. As the saying goes -- "Too much of a good thing ..."

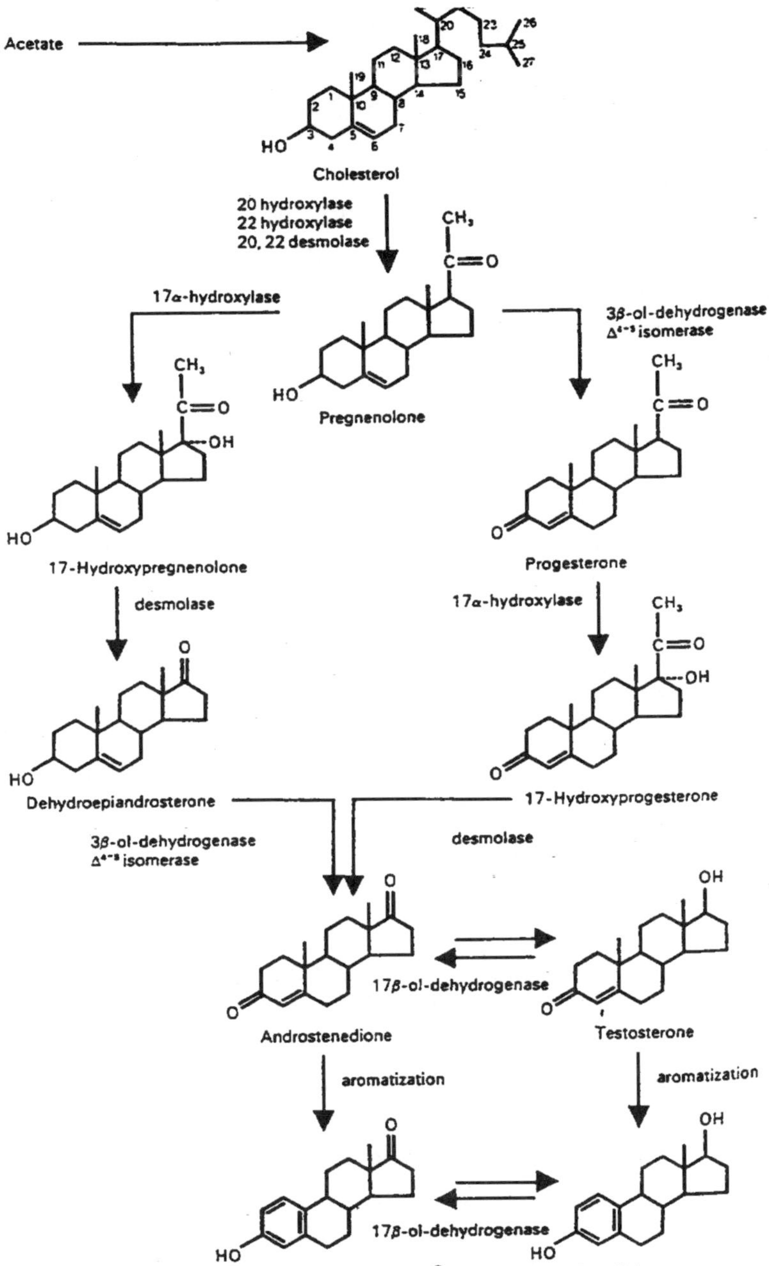
Acetate
Cholesterol
20 hydroxylase
22 hydroxylase
20, 22 desmolase
Pregnenolone
17α-hydroxylase
3β-ol-dehydrogenase
Δ4-5 isomerase
17-Hydroxypregnenolone
Progesterone
desmolase
17α-hydroxylase
Dehydroepiandrosterone
17-Hydroxyprogesterone
3β-ol-dehydrogenase
Δ4-5 isomerase
desmolase
Androstenedione
17β-ol-dehydrogenase
Testosterone
aromatization
aromatization
Estrone
17β-ol-dehydrogenase
Estradiol

Now this is a very complicated chemical scheme, yet this very complex set of reactions goes on daily in the **ovaries** and in the **testes**, and to a small extent as well in the **adrenal glands** of both sexes. The production of these three hormones depends upon pituitary control, as we have noted before, and when released into the blood for influence on other tissues, they are transported, connected to or attached to special proteins in the blood stream. They then enter at the cellular level through a special receptor mechanism. This is the receptor mechanism we mentioned. Once the hormones have been used in the target organ appropriately, they are again returned to the blood and transported to more tissues that are in need of them. Some hormones are unchanged when promoting or facilitating tissue reaction. They can be used again and again until destroyed by specific processes in the liver. Estrogen is usually transported to the liver for breakdown. In contrast, testosterone is most often broken down in the target organ cells. In either instance, the breakdown products are eliminated from the body in urine, bile and fecal waste.

All three of these hormones are in the bloodstream of males and females at all times. As we have noted, progesterone, testosterone, and estrogen are present in different concentrations in males and females, dependent upon physiologic need. Once again, all three are in free form in very small amounts, but the greatest amounts are bound to serum proteins and are released as the need is made known by the cells of the body. The transport to, and transport across some cell membranes, is intensely complex and is a tribute to the wonder, the mystery, and the phenomenal organization of our bodies. The biochemical reactions that take place are truly remarkable.

Generally destruction or breakdown of these hormones,

in the liver cells, is efficient and without harm to the individual. It is the damaged liver (from infection and/or substance abuse) that has a real problem with hormonal breakdown and disposal. A healthy liver manages these processes quite well.

Chapter 1 Overview

- Hormones are produced in special organs known as Endocrine Glands
- Hormones influence other organs and tissues to function
- The male hormone, testosterone comes from the testes and adrenal glands
- Hormones are vital in maintaining good health and activity

Chapter 2 The Effects of Estrogen in the Genetic Female

The young female, up to the average age of 12 years, has about the same body shape (habitus), the same voice pitch, the same daily organ system function, as does her young male counterpart. Her pituitary gland has been active, providing stimulus to other endocrine glands to continue development, growth, and normal physiology, but there has been no real influence on her reproductive organs. Usually between the ages of 10 and 13, a pituitary hormone we call a **gonadotropin** with influence on the ovaries, will start stimulating special cells in the ovaries to begin their cyclic activity in producing the sex hormone estrogen (estradiol). That gonadotropin is called **follicle stimulating hormone**. Once this interaction begins, the pituitary and the ovary will maintain a relationship, influencing each other in an ever recurrent cyclic manner for all of the reproductive years.

With the beginning of ovarian activity, only estrogen is produced. The responses it engenders are dramatic. This is the pubertal time for the female. During this phase, hair growth begins in the arm pits and the pubic area, fat stores are redistributed, and her body shape becomes very characteristically female. Her torso assumes more of the "hour glass" shape. Long bone growth is actually halted, and stature is fixed under the influence of estrogen. The skin and scalp hair change. Most notably, her breasts begin to develop having more size, volume and shape. On entering puberty she begins her journey into womanhood. After a year or so of these alterations, the pituitary gland exerts more of its influence upon the ovaries. Another gonadotropin, **luteinizing hormone**, is produced, stimulating those same special cells in the ovary to produce progesterone and to make eggs. This process, called **ovulation**, now allows her to be fertile -- she can now reproduce. She then has an instinctual drive to conceive. She may have had some uterine bleeding to this point (anovulatory periods), but now as she begins ovulatory function on a somewhat regular basis and she continues to ovulate, she will menstruate until her mid 40's or early 50's. At this time she will have a loss of ovarian activity **(menopause)** and a gradual and then eventually complete loss of production of estrogen and progesterone.

All through the years of estrogen production many other organ systems have benefited and have been maintained under the influence of estrogen. To give only one important example of estrogenic influence, consider the following: **Estrogen** is very much a part of the lipid, or fat metabolism in the female. It influences the levels of cholesterol in the blood, as well as the important transport substances for cholesterol, the lipoproteins **LDL** and **HDL**. These substances have a great deal to do with the development of arteriosclerosis, or atheromatous plaque formation in the arteries, particularly in the arteries of the h eart. Estrogen retards the development of this vessel disease. The genetic female develops cardiovascular disease at a much slower rate in her life while she is producing estrogen. This is in contrast to her male counterpart, who doesn't have such a protective mechanism in place.

All aspects of her femininity and continuing good health will be contributed to by her estrogen production. There comes a time in every female's life when she will begin to undergo changes in pituitary and ovarian function, with consequent changes in the making of estrogen and progesterone. As time progresses she moves into the menopausal phase of her life. She will make less and less estrogen and ovulate much more seldom with subsequent loss of fertility.

In addition, there is often a diminished libido, and eventually a loss altogether of her menstrual periods. As one looks at the aging female, there are very notable alterations in her skin and in her hair. There will be changes in the position and size of her breasts and distinct changes in subcutaneous fat storage and distribution throughout the body. Her bone metabolism will change and she then becomes susceptible to a condition known as **osteoporosis**. The danger of bone fracture increases with time because of this change in the bones, brought about by the loss of estrogen influence. Her stature and posture will reflect this as well. She becomes shorter and somewhat bent. Her cholesterol metabolism will be altered considerably, and she now becomes a candidate for blood vessel change and the development of heart disease. In fact, women well into menopause and beyond, experience the same changes in coronary artery disease that males experience at an earlier age. The mortality rates for women due to heart accident catches up to that of men who began this process some time before.

Chapter 2 Overview

- Estrogen is a hormone in the genetic female that is produced at puberty and continues to be functional until menopause
- Estrogen's influence is noted in the formation of the female body shape and in the maintenance of her bones plus a host of other systems
- Estrogen's involvement is necessary in many body functions to maintain the genetic female's good health and fertility

Chapter 3 The Effects of Testosterone in the Genetic Male

As stated before, the genetic male will have about the same body shape, voice pitch and daily organ function as does the young female, his counterpart. His pubertal development may be a little bit less active and slower to produce change than his female counterpart. However, once the pituitary begins stimulating the testes, first with the gonadotropin follicle-stimulating hormone, and eventually the second gonadotropin, luteinizing hormone, testicular development and production of testosterone and sperm cells will begin in earnest.

Along with a number of other influences, particularly growth hormone from the pituitary gland, the young male will now begin to grow in stature and to develop impressive shoulder musculature, chest and back. His muscle mass everywhere will increase considerably and muscle strength will be quite extraordinarily changed. His legs take on more bulk. His hands and feet grow. He develops a beard. Pubic and axillary (armpit) hair begin to become quite prominent, along with extremity hair.

Along with changes in other body tissues and organs, there is distinct change in the size of his **penis** and the **scrotum**. There is stimulus to the testes from the pituitary to develop sperm cells in specialized cells of the testes, and there is stimulus as well to the accessory sex organs, the **prostate** and **seminal vesicles** to contribute fluid, which will be the vehicle for the many thousands of sperm cells. This is known as the ejaculate.

As this young man continues to progress in puberty, he will have sudden and spontaneous penile erections and at night will have what are known as "wet dreams", wherein spontaneous ejection of that ejaculate takes place while asleep.

In addition to very great physical change, that young man now has a great deal of emotional alteration as well. He becomes quite aggressive and dominant in many of his dealings and attitudes. There will be moments of great quiet and mild depression along with spurts of real anger and aggression. As he moves further into his teens, he begins to think strongly about the females around him and his interest in sexual activity is heightened. There will be great need to prove his sexual prowess and it will be necessary to demonstrate, not only to himself but to his peers, success in sexual encounters. He may become intensely athletic. A great deal has to do with his environment and the stimulus of his peers. But his male attitude, behavior, and levels of success will have a great deal to do with hormone production.

As he continues through his late teens and into his third and fourth decade and beyond, his testosterone levels will stay quite elevated, generally not as much on a cyclic basis as estrogen is in the female. There is evidence that his testosterone levels will stay relatively high well into his 50's and even into his 60's and 70's. His potency and ability to be quite adequate and successful in his sexual activity may extend into older age. In time however, while **testosterone** levels stay elevated, his libido or sexual appetite may change notably. All through his life, testosterone has continued to maintain his skeletal system and his muscular vigor and strength. But one of the things that will not profit well because of **testosterone** production is his **cardiovascular** health. Androgenic substances, such as testosterone, have influence upon the development of arteriosclerosis in the arteries, and eventually changes due to lipid deposits in the walls of the arteries, particularly in the heart, will lead to changes in blood flow to the cardiac musculature, hence an ever progressive cardiac muscle deterioration and dysfunction will take place.

This process actually begins quite early in life, much earlier than it does in the genetic female, for she has some cardio-protective value from her estrogen production. Eventually in time, dependent upon the amount of exercise, the amount of tobacco use and whether or not obesity, hypertension and diabetes are existent as well, along with other factors inclusive of hereditary tendencies, the male individual, if no other disease or accident intervenes, will die of cardiovascular disease brought on in part by his testosterone production.

Chapter 3 Overview

- Testosterone is the essential hormone produced in the young male at puberty
- Testosterone will influence the male's body development and function throughout his life. Some of those functions are fertility, red blood cell production and lipid profile
- Testosterone, in spite of the many important functions and physiologic systems it maintains in a male's lifetime, can contribute to his death from cardiovascular disease

Chapter 4 The Doctor's Evaluation of You For a Masculinizing Program

Let's talk about the initial approach your physician will utilize in preparing you for the use of hormones.

Very probably, you are in excellent health, able to use a hormonal regimen with no intrusion or alteration in your health status. But you and your physician must be certain. Your doctor will want to make enquiry about your past medical and surgical history and will ask as well into various aspects of health, of disease occurrence and mode of death of various family members. This is very important. Certain disorders that tend to occur in families must be discussed. I refer to diseases such as hypertension, heart disease, particularly due to arteriosclerotic disease, diabetes, obesity, and liver disorders. You should be prepared before going into the doctor's office for that kind of inquiry, hence make appropriate investigation into your family history. Your doctor will also make inquiry into your alcohol, drug and tobacco use. You should know completely and be able to relate fully your own past medical and surgical experiences. If there is any obstetrical or gynecologic history of importance, this must also be a part of the enquiry. Menstrual irregularities, obstetrical experience, and gynecological infections will be a part of the information you should be prepared to give. There is good evidence in the medical literature that 25% of all preoperative F to M individuals have **ovarian cystic disease**, and that a significant number of this group have elevated levels of **androgens** (testosterone-like hormones) in their blood. Just what the significance of this may be is not completely clear. But it could account for some menstrual dysfunction in some individuals and it may be important that pelvic ultrasound study be done in the initial evaluation to determine whether or not ovarian cystic changes are present.

A thorough sexual activity history is important. It is wise, once again, to review these things before going to your doctor's office, so that you know all of this for ready discussion.

Your physical exam should be a very complete one. Your doctor should do a complete evaluation of your eye grounds. The retinal area, or the back of the eye, can tell a great deal about certain types of diseases, or the potential for developing them. He or she should conduct also a careful neurologic exam and inspect the lower extremities for vein incompetency and pulses. Your doctor should examine the thyroid area to be sure that there are no enlargements. Close attention to blood pressure and weight are very important. Blood pressure measurements in each arm and weight recording are essentials not only the initial evaluation but in every examination thereafter. Evaluation of your heart and lungs is necessary and your abdomen must be examined to be sure that there are no enlargements, or any change in liver size.

Evaluation of your breasts and a discussion of proper self-breast examination is necessary. A very thorough pelvic and rectal examination must be done as well. A pap smear and appropriate cultures when needed are also most important.

Baseline blood evaluations will be done to insure good health and to detect any alteration once the hormonal regimen is started. General studies include the basic profile done to rule out blood cell abnormalities, and evaluation of kidney function and liver activity are important. It will be necessary that your doctor conduct a lipid profile which includes cholesterol, triglycerides, HDL and LDL determinations. Evaluation of the thyroid is done with specific blood tests, and serum electrolytes as well as serum calcium, phosphorus and blood glucose are equally important. A urinalysis will also be done and urine cultures should they be indicated, will be obtained.

While it may not be necessary to repeat some major hormone level studies in the blood beyond the initial evaluation—the **pituitary gonadotropins (follicle stimulating hormones, luteinizing hormone levels)** prolactin levels, blood estrogen (Estradiol) and testosterone levels are important baseline studies.

Special studies as are indicated, relative to general health concerns, are of course part of this initial baseline evaluative approach. Some of these studies may be necessary to repeat in the monitoring to come, once on hormones. Special studies relative to heart, liver, vein competency, various scan techniques, EKG's, cardiac stress testing and the like, all must be a part of the initial or ongoing assessment of your general health as your doctor feels it important. Your doctor's responsibility involves not only just prescribing contragender hormonal therapy but also maintaining your overall health and being aware whenever changes that are adverse, take place. While most transgendered individuals can use contragender hormones quite safely, a few will have changes in their health status that are adverse and for some, these may be very serious. They must be identified and managed appropriately.

This means that you have just as much responsibility to

keep your periodic monitoring appointments with your physician as he or she has in scheduling them and conducting them properly.

Chapter 4 Overview

- It is essential to have an initial history taken and a thorough physical examination with complete laboratory studies before a masculinizing hormonal regimen is started
- The initial studies provide a valuable baseline to compare with the periodic examinations (monitoring) to follow while the masculinizing regimen is in progress
- To omit monitoring risks one's health and may hinder the effectiveness of the masculinizing process

Chapter 5 The Masculinizing Process

"Tissue response and time are just as important to consider as is the dose and the hormone."

One concept that is important to emphasize when treating the genetic female with masculinizing hormones is that you and your physician are really tampering with systems that have been in place for all of your life. The genetic female has factors in motion to account for her physical appearance that are genetic as well as hormonal. She is lighter, smaller, and shorter. Her facial features are finer, her skeletal development quite different in some respects. She will always be, even when treated vigorously with testosterone, a small individual, particularly if she does not gain large amounts of weight and remains quite lean. Her genetic inheritance is biologically female.

Another concept to keep in mind is that tissue response and time will bring to the individual virtually all that is to be accomplished for that particular individual. There really is no shortcut to alteration of physical characteristics.

Next, I advise you that while routes of administration of testosterone for the FTM individual are both by mouth and by intramuscular injection, the latter is thought to be the better approach. Although, just recently, a transdermal system (skin patch) has been developed—a better one than previously available skin patches for delivering testosterone, no conclusive studies for the FTM person are yet reported to the medical literature. The research work done thus far is only on genetic men whose testicular function is underactive (hypogonadal). In them the masculinizing results using a patch are excellent. Studies for the FTM will be reported without doubt. The outlook for those using this skin patch known as Androderm seems promising as well. Liver involvement is lessened by injection and transdermal routes and more importantly, the effects are experienced in a more even manner.

In the genetic female, the expected responses to **testosterone** are these:

Menstrual function

On an adequate regimen, half of those taking the hormone will have no **menses** after three months. Almost all will lose their menstrual function within six months of hormone use. A small number will have some menstrual activity or intermittent spotting and require alterations in dosage or addition of an oral progestational agent, such as **Provera** or **Aygestin**. There are distinct changes that take place in the lining of the uterus to eliminate menstrual activity.

Voice Pitch

Testosterone, when circulating in adequate serum concentration, will change the thickness and function of the vocal cords for virtually all using it. Occasional individuals will not respond as fully as others, but for most, the voice pitch will lower into the male range. The change is complete enough to make the individual's voice masculine, not only in person to person conversation but on the telephone as well. The **FTM** individual will not be able to sing in higher ranges as before. All this is quite dramatic and quite **irreversible.**

Hair growth

It takes time, but distinct patterns of hair growth take place. On the face in several years, a full beard is virtually a reality. Chest and extremity hair growth will be stimulated. The extent varies from one to another, but if hair follicles exist in an area, the hair growth will be evident over time. Paradoxically for some, male pattern baldness may take place as well.

Muscular Development

Because of the anabolic or tissue-building property of testosterone, muscle mass will develop and muscle strength will increase. An occasional individual complains of extremity and joint pain, thought to be due to the strain of increased muscle mass on the tendons and their attachments to bone. The individual who exercises and lifts weights will have even more development. Some anabolic steroids produce more muscle mass than do others.

Clitoral Change

The clitoris will enlarge and for some the length may be quite notable, up to 6 cm. Again, tissue response is the essential factor, but this is a very striking change for those who experience it. (refer to page 28)

Certain changes will not take place:

Skeletal Alteration and Torso Shape

These will not change for the FTM individual. Genetic females are generally smaller, built with a slender, lighter appearance. There will be no skeletal changes in the chest cage or the pelvic region when taking testosterone. The height of the individual remains the same. Estrogen production at puberty closes the epiphysial growth plates located at the ends of long bones. Hands and feet will remain small and facial features will not change in their delicateness. The individual will be a small appearing male.

Breast changes

While some distinct cellular changes in various structures of the breast are changed and perhaps with weight reduction, fat storage will diminish, the breasts will not become appreciably smaller. The small-breasted individual will be at a greater advantage, certainly, than the full-breasted genetic female when it comes time for top surgery. Large breasts in genetic females may become somewhat pendulous and dependent with time. Binding makes that dependency even more evident. However, for some binding, is very important until their breasts are removed when the male chest appearance is created by a surgeon. Many surgeons advise against binding due to the changes that binding induces, making surgical results less than optimal.

Chapter 5 Overview

- Expect good progress when you are on an adequate contragender hormone regimen, but don't look for unrealistic and unobtainable results.
- With **testosterone** use, **menses** will disappear within 6 months. If this doesn't occur talk with your physician
- With **testosterone** use, voice pitch lowers, facial and body hair increases, emotional changes will be experienced
- Many body systems will be influenced by **testosterone** as they are in the genetic male-hence the need for proper and regular medical evaluations

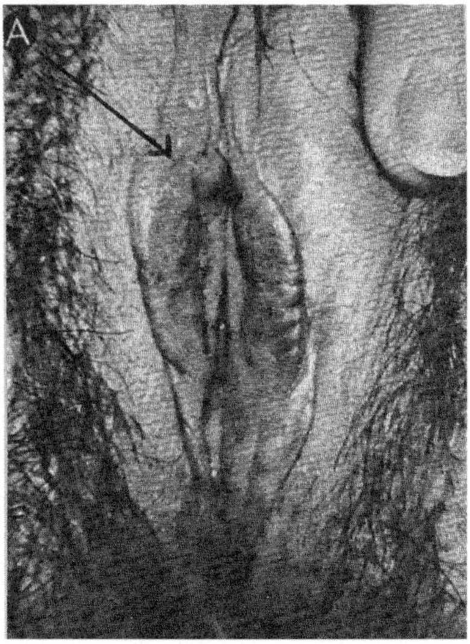

Figure 1.
The Normal Clitoris

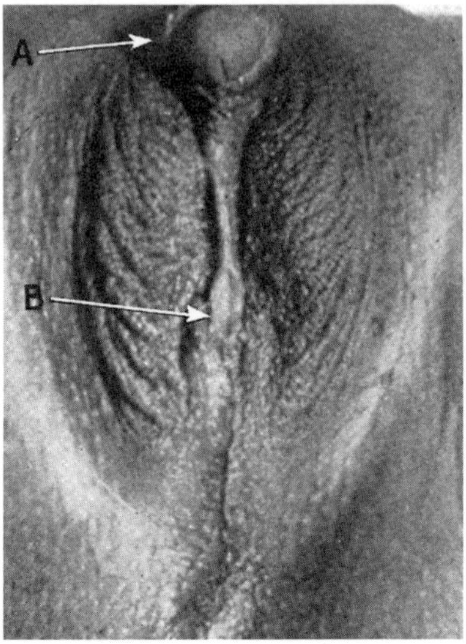

Figure 2.

A - The enlarged clitoris under testosterone influence

B - Urethral opening obscured —very small vaginal opening

Chapter 6 Annoyances and Problems On Testosterone

The annoyances that are often encountered when using a masculinizing hormone:

Fluid Retention

Peripheral edema or fluid retention for some may be a very difficult problem, especially with lower extremity vein incompetency. The tendency for sodium and water retention overall is a problem that may require the use of diuretics. Diuretics are medications that stimulate the kidneys to pass more urine. Sodium and potassium are passed with the urine, hence, tests for electrolyte levels in the blood may be needed periodically. With difficulty in mobilizing retained fluid in the body or the extremities, compressive hosiery (support hose) may be needed and sometimes sodium in the diet may need to be restricted. Some of the weight increase on this therapy is certainly due to this problem.

Weight Increase

Even for those who are slim, beginning testosterone can create weight increase difficulties. For those already overweight or obese, this can be a major complication and great care must be taken to become calorie conscious and make every effort to lose weight and then maintain it. A plan for diet sensibility and weight loss with real attention to calorie counting may be a constant way of life. While fluid retention and increased muscle mass can be a part of the weight gain, eating habits must be reviewed to control this problem. Excess weight can contribute to other health problems and can lead to serious difficulties with hypertension and cardiovascular disease. It all begins at the grocery store. Proper purchases and preparation are then in order-all of it associated with calorie counting and fat and cholesterol content in mind.

Skin Changes

The vigorous influence of testosterone on all the glands and structures in the skin accounts for a considerable number of **FTM** individuals complaining of **acne**. Intensive facial care may be needed using good cleansing practices and topical acne creams and medications. There may even be a need for antibiotic therapy for a few individuals. Give attention to this difficulty and take the steps to rid yourself of skin infections and to maintain a good complexion. Whether you wear a beard or not, treat your skin with appropriate attention and care.

On a masculinizing hormonal therapy regimen there is a potential for much more serious problems:

Blood Cell Changes

Red blood and white blood cells are developed in the marrow of our bones. It is here that testosterone exerts its affect upon red blood cell production. In fact, some people afflicted with certain forms of anemia and leukemia are given testosterone-like medications to stimulate the "manufacture" of red blood cells. Some **FTM** individuals when on testosterone may demonstrate changes in their blood hemoglobin and in the quantity of the red blood cells beyond the normal range. This condition is called polycythemia. Management of this will depend on the severity of the change brought to this blood building system by the hormone therapy. Alterations in the testosterone regimen, in addition to the standard treatment for this condition, may be needed.

Liver Changes

Liver enzyme elevations will be noted in a significant number of hormone users. Generally, they are transient elevations dropping to acceptable levels as hormone use continues. Levels that are too high will necessitate interruption of the testosterone regimen and subsequent evaluation of the liver. Without discovery of significant liver disease, the regimen could be started again, but at lower dose and with very gradual increases to accomplish appropriate physical changes. If the patient's history and baseline study of liver function indicates that there could be any antecedent liver problem due to alcohol use or infection, you may not be a candidate from the start for testosterone therapy. Occasional subjects will not have a known history and they have persistently elevated enzymes even after the testosterone is stopped. This must be studied and the reasons for liver dysfunction then must be discovered. A monitoring of liver health is all important throughout the individual's lifetime while using hormones, so be prepared for periodic testing of this organ's competency.

Hypertension

Mild **blood pressure** elevation can be made worse in an individual with existing hypertension. Also, a hypertension potential can become evident when testosterone is used. The degree of hypertension and the response to hypertensive therapy will determine whether the testosterone dose is to be continued, to be moderated or stopped altogether. The concern is that, over time, testosterone use may hasten vessel arteriosclerotic disease and thereby induce heart disease. **Hypertension** has an effect upon the heart as well. The two in combination, heart vessel disease and heart changes due to elevated blood pressure, can cause very **severe** health problems. Your physician must be very watchful and ready to treat hypertension vigorously, even to the point of stopping hormone therapy. Worsening of preexistent hypertension must be approached with a very appropriate medical plan and that plan must work or the whole regimen must be stopped.

Lipid Profile

For some masculinizing hormones can cause alterations in serum cholesterol, triglycerides and the lipoproteins **HDL** and **LDL.** There is the fear that if these substances become so altered or out of proper ratio, they will eventually exert influence upon the blood vessels (arteries) and their function, leading to coronary artery and heart disease. The gender team at the Free University of Amsterdam, Netherlands, has a moderately large number of **FTM** individuals they have followed for some time (over 1000 individuals both MTF and FTM). In a recent report, they found that on a testosterone regimen both HDL and HDL 2 cholesterol, fractions of serum cholesterol in circulation returning to the liver, known also as "good" cholesterol, are lowered by this therapy. It is known that lowered amounts of these two substances in the blood are linked to the development of heart disease. This is particularly so with the **HDL 2** fraction. What this means is that more study is needed to clarify this research data, and the impact of lowered HDL on the heart of an FTM person. More study is needed in the **FTM** population in specific to determine just what this means in a population whose basic genetic profile is female and who are being rendered estrogen deficit through medication and surgery.

If an improper lipid profile develops, steps should be taken to improve these laboratory determinations and halt any detrimental process leading to ill health. Diet, exercise, cessation of smoking and appropriate medication when indicated, could be in the picture. Whether testosterone is to be continued, modified or stopped depends upon patient response to the regimen instituted for an abnormal lipid profile. If improvement does not take place, the hormonal regimen is to be stopped.

Cardiovascular Disease

Candidates for testosterone should be selected with no hint of cardiovascular concern in their baseline evaluations. If the cardiovascular system is suspect, proper evaluation is mandatory ***before*** any hormone is begun. If cardiovascular disease develops during therapy, the hormonal regimen is halted and the patient evaluated fully with the thought that hormones may or may not be used again. There is one report in the medical literature regarding cardiovascular accident in an **FTM** individual on testosterone. The loss of cardio-protective value of estrogen along with the concern of premature cardiovascular disease while on testosterone has made some researchers speak of this potential in the medical literature. In theory, it is all very possible and more time and more studies are needed. The physician monitoring the **FTM** individual must be aware of this concern for each and every patient on a testosterone regimen.

Two additional considerations must be kept in mind. The first is phlebitis and the second has to do with emotional change.

Phlebitis (vein inflammation) This is a relatively uncommon complaint for the FTM individual. It is a serious one nonetheless, and it can't be emphasized enough. This condition is an infection principally but it can be associated with blood clot formation. When it does, should the clot(s) break off or detach from the vein wall, it will travel through the circuit of veins to the heart and then to the lungs. This is known as **embolism**. **Embolism** can be so severe as to cause death. This is a very serious disease, concerning enough to give you some additional details about it.

Your physician can acquaint you with some of the signs and symptoms of **phlebitis**, but here is something to help in your understanding of this condition.

To begin with-there are two vein systems in our bodies - a superficial and a deep one. They interconnect and they function to bring blood that carries carbon dioxide and metabolic waste to our excretory organs for disposal and to the heart and lungs for oxygen replenishment. They can become inflamed and blood clots can develop. Both conditions are serious and its when the deep system has clots in it that embolism can take place. The clots can break or detach and go through the circuits to the heart to eventually lodge in the lungs. The degree of clot transport to the lungs determines the severity of the embolic episode. When slight or moderate in the smaller lung veins, the symptoms are chest pain and breathing difficulties. When the blood clots to the lungs are many or large or lodge in major veins, then the condition can be catastrophic leading to death. Inflammation in the veins of lower extremities or the pelvic veins of the deep system give pain and often fever along with sudden development of foot, ankle and lower leg swelling.

There is immobility and difficulty in walking. Abdomen pain can take place before any chest pains begin. The inflammation and/or clotting of the deep system can be subtle and progressive giving time to allow accurate diagnosis. It can, however, be sudden and overwhelming particularly after trauma or surgery.

Infection in the superficial systems takes place most of

the time in the lower extremities, one leg or both. It very seldom has embolism associated although clotting can and often does take place. The lower limb becomes painful, swollen and reddened. There may be a streak along the course of a superficial vein in the skin. It hurts to walk. Notably complaints may happen overnight or even over several hours.

The diagnosis of phlebitis in either system requires an immediate and often prolonged interruption of the masculinizing medical regimen. Treatment will be based on the system involved and the extent of the process in the estimate of the physician by physical examination and laboratory study. Other aspects of underlying health status must be taken into consideration as well.

Your physician must be in constant watchfulness for the development of this disturbing complication, and you should have some instruction to look for early preliminary signs if such a process is in place. Sometimes however, phlebitis is rather insidious and you may only have discomfort and swelling in one leg without demonstrating too much more in the way of complaint. Anything that is indicative of change in the way your lower extremities feel or appear, certainly should be reported to your doctor.

Emotional Changes

For some, there may be no emotional alterations whatever. However, a great number of individuals do report times when they have extraordinary amounts of energy and aggressiveness, and it may be coupled with outbursts of anger and erratic or exaggerated response to ordinary situations and stress. Some individuals even report inordinate amounts of rage.

Overall, many of these kinds of responses take place

while early in hormonal therapy, although some note that these feelings are intensified just after their injection of medication. In time, these outbursts of anger and emotional upset lessen. However, some individuals still report moments wherein they have extraordinary amounts of energy and may even have extraordinary amounts of heightened sexual interest. They may have need for sexual outlet in order to control these feelings. In time however, most individuals make very positive adjustments to their medication and outbursts of anger and emotional upset lessen. While they have many of the same pressures with family and the workplace as does every other individual, their abilities to cope and to adjust seem to be much more positive. Overall, the fact that an individual taking hormones is well on his way towards contragender change can make him much happier and a more productive individual.

Chapter 6 Overview

- Annoyances while not life-threatening often occur with a contragender hormonal regimen
- Serious even life threatening problems and complications can occur on a contragender program using testosterone.
- Be certain that your physician possesses adequate medical knowledge in contragender hormonal care and treatment
- If you believe that your health care professional lacks adequate knowledge in treatment and management—change professionals
- Periodic evaluation by a competent physician is vital in order to avoid or to possibly correct potential problems or serious concerns on a masculinizing regimen

Chapter 7 Medications Commonly Used in the Masculinization of the FTM Individual

To be sure, there are a great number of oral medications available, and some doctors are still prescribing them. Some of those oral preparations can lead to much more difficult problems and complications. In addition, the oral approach is not as effective or efficient as the regimen which uses intramuscular injection. Oral medication is not always completely absorbed from the gastrointestinal tract. Testosterone placed into the blood stream directly with injection is far more efficient. There is a new approach now available to the FTM individual. This is the recently developed Transdermal System or skin patch known as Androderm.

Because not many FTM individuals choose to use oral medication—I will not list the many products available. Some are Testosterone-like products that induce masculinizing change primarily. Others have strong Anabolic properties in addition to their testosterone effect. By this it is meant, these steroids can be used to build muscle mass and thereby create a very athletic body. These latter products introduce a new factor in the FTM process one that for most is not necessary and for many not safe. Close supervision by a knowledgeable physician is essential. It's a form of therapy that doesn't belong in the regimen of most.

The most common injectable medications in common usage are these:

Testosterone Enanthate (known also as **Delatestryl**)

— This medication is given by injection every two to four weeks in doses of 100-400 mg. depending upon the individual's well being and clinical response.

Testosterone Propionate (known as **Neo-hombreol**) — This medication is also given by injection every two to four weeks in doses of 100-200 mg. and dose elevations are very much related to the individual's comfort and clinical response.

Testosterone Cypionate (known as **Depo-Testosterone**) — This medication is given every two to four weeks by injection in doses that range from 100-400 mg. Adjustments in dosage are made with clinical response and individual comfort.

Transdermal System (known as **Androderm**) — Men whose testes don't produce adequate amounts of the male hormone, Testosterone, are known as hypogonadal. Skin patches had been developed for use in this type of male patient before the Androderm Patch, but they were not always the most efficient in transferring the hormone through the skin to the circulating blood. In addition, they could not be placed just anywhere on the body or the extremities. They had to be placed on the scrotum where many blood vessels existed in the skin—far more than in other places. Those patch systems were a poor choice for the FTM person who had to place the skin patch on or near to the labia or on the inner thigh. This provided poor hormone transfer through the skin.

In contrast, Androderm can be placed anywhere on the body or extremities. Passage through the skin of Testosterone is very efficient and the blood concentrations are in the proper range as in healthy genetic men. The technique requires that either one or two patches are applied nightly every 24 hours. The drawbacks are few;

local skin irritation and rash are complaints for about 10% of users. Headaches are experienced by 5%. An additional drawback is cost although in time it could be expected that the cost will be lowered. I would emphasize that you need to exercise patience. During this time of therapy, you should be watching very carefully your weight and incorporating into your diet practices and habits that can be helpful and appropriate to maintaining your good health.

Some individuals have reported that the introduction of vegetables, particularly green vegetables and in specific broccoli, is very helpful in eliminating many emotional upsets. Overall, however, a very definite sense of well being should come to the individual who is using testosterone successfully and comfortably. Any experiences that seem inappropriate or an interference with comfortable daily activity should be reported to your doctor.

Chapter 7 Overview

- Never exceed recommended dosages. To do so risks your health and your life
- Patience and time are important ingredients during the contragender regimen
- Individuals respond differently to hormonal treatment. This variability is based on your own biologic make-up, not necessarily the contragender regimen
- Regimens and dosages can be modified to accomplish optimal results on the advice of your physician. Safety should not be sacrificed and should always be kept in mind

Chapter 8 Follow-Up Monitoring--Periodic Reexamination and Laboratory

Evaluations

For a while your doctor may require that you come to the office frequently for evaluation of your health and to review the efficiency of your hormonal regimen. Those visits may seem to be often for a time, but certainly with a measure of stability in your reaction to medication, and with the assurance that all is progressing in a comfortable manner, those visits can be spaced considerably. In time you can be taught to use injectable medication yourself, thereby lessening cost and the number of visits. Regardless whether injections or a skin patch your physician needs to see you to evaluate your progress. Physical changes will need evaluation and laboratory studies will be necessary with those visits. Changes in the regimen may be instituted depending on what each visit reveals to you and your doctor. Your doctor should keep good records regarding your progress.

Generally, by the time you have reached the second year of treatment, evaluation and laboratory studies can be extended to twice a year and should continue as such for the next two or three years, depending upon whether you are a candidate for reassignment surgery, or whether you are delaying for any number of personal reasons. During that time, assessments of the hormonal regimen are made and decided upon by you and your physician. Keep in mind that even after major reassignment surgery is done, monitoring must continue on a periodic basis usually once each year, dependent upon your physical health and freedom from illness.

If prior to phalloplasty you have had breast removal and hysterectomy, with removal of both ovaries, then you don't need periodic mammography and pelvic examination with Pap Smear. Generally, by the time you come to these surgical experiences, voice change and hair growth should have progressed very well and a maintenance medical regimen will have been instituted. Your interval physical examinations need not be extensive by this time in your transition. However, they should always include weight, blood pressure determination (both arms), evaluation of the legs in the appropriate places for pulse presence and equality, and vein competency and a quick listen to the heart. If you have not had reassignment surgery or breast removal, then breast examination by your doctor, a pelvic with Pap Smear when it is appropriate in time must also be performed. You should also be conducting self-breast examinations every 4-6 weeks.(See Chapter 9 on Self-breast examination.)

You may believe that mammography is no longer needed once you have started testosterone therapy. I don't agree! When you are using testosterone, it is true that it suppresses ovarian activity and estrogen levels in the blood decline notably. Keep in mind, however, that not all breast cancers are estrogen dependent. There are only a small percentage of genetic females wherein there is a family of breast cancer. These cancers are developed through genetic transmission, and they can progress even without estrogen stimulus. Until the breasts are removed then self-breast examination and periodic mammography must still be done. Only after hysterectomy which includes removal of the cervix can pelvic examination with Pap Smear be omitted from your periodic evaluations.

Laboratory studies should include an evaluation of your lipid profile, liver function studies, and a complete blood cell count with differential and indices. A blood testosterone determination showing how near to the male range your medication is assisting you, can be done periodically. Dependent upon prior experience in your medical health, and previous findings in your electrocardiographic studies, a careful and thorough cardiac profile should be considered at periodic intervals.

A very important measure to record is clitoral length. This can be done by you in private reporting to the physician what changes have occurred, or measurement can be taken at the time of the pelvic exam. These measurements should be recorded as well. (See Chapter 9.)

There should be inquiry about health factors in both you and members of your family since you were last seen. It is very important to include in discussions with your physician, alcohol use, smoking and weight concerns and your progress in managing these areas. Some discussion about emotional health is necessary and all this should be a part of the record-keeping, along with notations regarding stress or other psychosocial concerns. It is necessary that this data be exchanged with your mental health-care therapist or counselor and eventually with the surgeon who will be entering the picture in the future.

Chapter 8 Overview

- Periodic monitoring CANNOT be stressed enough
- Acquaint yourself with the recommended monitoring process and inform your physician that you want it to be followed
- Arrange for your medical records to be transferred when necessary and shared with any medical or health care professional who cares for you. Information exchanged between all of your care providers means better care for you

Chapter 9 Clitoral and Breast Self-Examinations

Clitoral Examination and Measurement

To measure the clitoris may be a little difficult. You may have to position yourself with a mirror and use a wooden or metal ruler that has measurements in centimeters (cms.) Don't push the ruler into the tissue too firmly and always place the ruler along the under surface of the clitoris to read the measurement. If the measurement of the clitoris is too difficult to read or too inconsistent from one exam to another, it will be necessary for another to do it -perhaps your partner or your doctor.

Self-Breast Examination

The incidence of serious breast disease --malignancy for the genetic female on a masculinizing hormonal regimen is not known. In addition to the possibility of cancer, benign breast disease can take place in your breast. When you have top surgery, then the need for self-breast examination ceases. But until then, it is still vital to continue this evaluation. Thickening, cysts and strange collections or buildup of tissue can develop and it is important to detect them and bring attention of these to your physician for accurate evaluation. Hence, I strongly urge you to learn the technique of self-breast examination described below and to conduct it once, every month, on a specific date or day.

In time, your awareness as to what are the usual findings in your own breasts becomes very accurate. The technique is not difficult. There are no shortcuts and thoroughness is important.

The technique is as follows —Lying down in supine position (on your back,) you will examine the left breast with the right hand, the right breast with the left hand. If you are full-breasted, it helps a little to place a pillow at your back with its inner margin just up to and in the length of the spine, thereby tipping you somewhat. Hence, the pillow is to the right side of your back and spine to examine the right breast, and the pillow is placed to the left side of your back and spine to examine the left breast. This keeps the breast on the front of the chest wall and tends to flatten it there. The pillow should not be overly thick. This technique allows you to feel deeply into the breast tissue. When the breast tissue is thick or dependent (as it is when you stand or sit to examine) you can miss significant changes that are deep in the breast tissue.

Now for the right breast. Pillow in place, you will raise the right arm over your head to put the breast on a stretch, and with the fingers of your left hand extended, you feel deeply into the right breast in a rotary motion covering all quadrants of the breast, moving from the periphery to the center of the breast, the nipple area. You feel the areola and nipple region completely as well. Once you have covered all the breast in this way, then you draw the extended left hand fingers across the breast, covering it all once again, in a stroking manner. This gives you two ways to evaluate the breast tissue: a) with deep point pressure and b) with a drawing or pulling of the fingers over the breast to detect any enlargements you may not have felt with the deep pressure. Now, if anything seems different or unusual, you repeat the above maneuvers to clarify or to confirm.

Changing the pillow placement, you raise the left arm above your head and with your right hand, examine the left breast the very same way.

I stress that you lie down to examine, for when sitting in front of a mirror or standing in the shower as many women are taught to examine, your breast is compact and dense. The breast tissue is dependent and firm, not allowing as full an evaluation of it as you can if it is a thinner organ with the chest wall firmly behind it. You can miss a tumor or growth when it is small and in early stages, when you do not lie down to examine.

In time, you will become very aware of any changes taking place in your breasts. Any change in the normal architecture becomes evident earlier with repetition and careful observation. Take the time to be thorough and be mindful of the need to always examine your breasts.

Chapter 10 Questions Commonly Asked

1. Once I start testosterone, do I have to worry about any gynecological or breast cancer developing?

There are no studies on just what cancer incidences are in the Transgendered FTM person to date. The suspicion is that cervical and breast cancer development in the FTM using testosterone are either the same or perhaps lower than the genetic female not taking testosterone. We need a well-controlled study to determine accurately the incidence. It must be stressed that the need to continue doing monthly self-breast exams and routine mammography and pelvic/pap smear examinations is most necessary. Cancer of the lungs because of smoking will be the same or perhaps increased because a considerable number of FTM individuals do smoke. Other cancers will likely not change incidence.

2. Is it more urgent that I quit smoking now that I am on testosterone?

Yes. The smoking link to Lung Cancer is now without question no matter what the tobacco companies say! The incidence of lung cancer in women who smoke has increased in the past decade and is in direct proportion to increased tobacco use in the female population. Non-malignant but none the less, life-threatening pulmonary diseases are also on the increase in these women. Another very real concern is the link between smoking and heart disease. It is a very established fact that they are related. And this should cause a FTM on testoster-

one a great concern. When we think of the possible development of heart disease in testosterone using (and estrogen deficient) genetic females—smoking as an added factor to this process is alarming! Which is it to be? Tobacco or testosterone? For good health and life expectancy, there shouldn't be both.

3. Can I develop sexually transmitted disease on testosterone?

The hormonal regimen will not change your susceptibility to these diseases. In fact, your selection of partner(s) is the primary concern in developing diseases from sexual contact. There is a distinct and alarming increase in HIV positivity and AIDS in the lesbian population within the last five years. Women are transmitting this very serious disease to women. Herpes is also transmitted in same sex relationships. Male hormone use actually has nothing to do with this problem.

4. Can I conceive a baby when I take testosterone by either male-female intercourse, artificial insemination or in virtro fertilization?

The probabilities are exceedingly small. The correct hormones in proper ratios must be present and their influence on the uterus must be appropriate to the process. Even with fertilization of the egg—implantation in the uterus won't take place and if it did, it would not develop for lack of the appropriate hormone climate. Male hormones must be stopped and there's no guarantee that normal ovarian function would be re-established especially if therapy had been in place for some time.

5. Can I expect my sex drive to change on Testosterone?

Yes. Libido and sexual performance both increase once you begin a contragender hormonal regimen. There may be wide swings in both with injection therapy.

6. Once I have all of my surgery, will I need to use testosterone any longer?

Yes. Testosterone in some kind of regimen will be needed for all of your lifetime unless a medical complication of serious nature demands interruption. The dosage might be lowered but should be monitored periodically.

7. Is it really necessary to have all the testing suggested? Not all doctors order the tests so why are they important?

Doctors who don't monitor your health in the correct ways with examinations and laboratory studies are playing with your health. These tests are important to gather information about your well-being and to monitor any possible changes that could affect it. If you don't insist on proper evaluations—you are jeopardizing your health.

8. How long will it take to have the full effects of hormones take place in my body?

Some physiologic systems will change quickly with therapy. Menses could stop completely in three months time. Complete voice deepening may take two years though some change is notable at six months. Extremity hair could take several years to be profuse and baldness maybe be evident within a year's time.

9. Is there any danger to interrupting my hormone therapy for several months at a time?

There could be individuals who have underlying heart disease or hypertension (overt or potential) which could place stress on the many mechanisms that regulate the blood vessels and the heart. Remember, there are no worthwhile studies as yet in the medical literature that report testosterone therapy in genetic females and its influence on their cardiovascular health.

10. I want to use testosterone and masculinize fully but I don't want phalloplasty just now and maybe not ever. Is that all right?

Yes it is! Health care professionals are aware of this attitude in the FTM community. They recognize that hormonal therapy and top surgery may be the only approaches many want in their contragender living. Metaidoioplasty (freeing of the clitoral hood) might be considered but phalloplasty may not even be in the planning. They not only recognize this attitude but many doctors are accepting to it.

11. I'm overweight now and about to start my testosterone medication. What can I expect?

You will be wise to lose the excess weight now before the regimen is started. Do whatever is necessary to accomplish this for without doubt whatever your eating habits are now, they are incorrect and they won't be at all easy to change once you start your therapy. Better to delay for a time, while you adopt new practices and lose weight. Masculinizing hormonal therapy will make it much harder for you to do so.

12. I've heard that maybe I'm at a greater risk for heart disease because I use testosterone. Is this true?

To the best of our knowledge at this time, testosterone tends to facilitate heart disease and estrogen is protective against it. Both hormones take part in our cholesterol metabolism. Again, testosterone can create problems for the levels of the various components of the lipid profile thereby accelerating arteriosclerosis. Estrogen slows that process. It is easy to believe that taking estrogen away and placing testosterone into your physiology will make you more vulnerable to heart problems. More study on this subject is necessary.

13. I've heard about mood swings and sometimes rages that some experience on testosterone. How can these be avoided?

Up to now, those taking injections of testosterone report their very labile emotions are most difficult just at injection and for a time thereafter. This implies that a "jolt" of hormone is responsible and that peak blood levels are the cause. If this is so, than a more controlled infusion of hormone by way of a Transdermal system could be a way to avoid such emotional outbursts with less "peaks and valleys" in testosterone levels in the blood.

14. I've never had complexion problems or acne before the start of testosterone. Now it is quite pronounced. What gives here?

Testosterone activates and stimulates the many glands in the skin particularly on the face, neck and shoulders, to produce more sweat and sebaceous material. Bacteria on the skin get into those glands and find a "home" there. The glands become infected—in some cases se-

verely so. This process will quiet down but in the meantime a visit or two to a dermatologist may be necessary.

15. Will testosterone use shrink my breasts?

No. While the estrogen stimulus that maintained them is now gone, testosterone doesn't alter the glandular or ductual structures to any extent. Fat storage in the breast will diminish with weight loss but surgery is the only way to "shrink" your breasts.

16. I understand from others that I could develop some male pattern baldness. I know that this helps to authenticate my male appearance but how much might take place?

There is no way to predict how much hair loss and balding could take place, if any at all. You will have to look at all the methods that men consider for hair loss should you encounter this annoyance.

17. If I keep my ovaries even with the phalloplasty operation-will I have any protection against heart disease?

The ovaries will become totally inactive and dormant. It's the estrogen they produce that is believed to be cardioprotective. No estrogen—no protection. It seems to me that psychologically you will want them removed. Cystic ovarian diseases if they develop could create problems because of pain or potential rupture.

18. Will my clitoris growth be great enough to penetrate my partner?

Testosterone can stimulate clitoral size to as much as 6 cm or just a little under 2.5 inches in some individuals. This is certainly notable change. The organ will retain it's sensitivity and the sexual experience will be exciting and satisfying for you and your partner. Penetration, however, will be only minimal at best.

19. I want to develop my body and increase my muscle mass. What must I do?

Certain testosterone products will assist you in this but the therapy may not be appropriate for some because of the real stress to many physiologic systems. You must be evaluated closely by your doctor while on such a program. Exercise and weight lifting can help greatly in developing that very athletic look. And it's safer!

20. I want lots of hair growth on my face, chest, arms and legs. When will it happen?

To some extent everyone will experience notable changes in hair patterns and growth. Just how much can't be predicted. The capacity of the hair follicles in your skin over the face and other areas to react to the hormonal stimulus is familial.

21. I'm going to wait for a time before I undergo phalloplasty. I want my uterus, tubes and ovaries removed now, however. My mind tells me it's the thing to do. What will it do to my health?

For your emotional health, it should be a real plus. For your physical health, it could remove a potential for uterine disease as serious as cancer and for ovarian disease as disturbing and cumbersome as cystic disease.

Definitions

Anabolic - A building up of tissue i.e.: increased muscle mass under the influence of male hormone.

Androgenic - Any substance that mimics or is similar in activity to testosterone.

Arteriosclerosis - A thickening of the wall of an artery with cholesterol, fat, blood cells and other constituents. Also know as atheromatous plaque disease and hardening of the arteries.

Cardiovascular - The combination of heart and blood vessel artery i.e. disease affecting both.

Diuretic - A medication taken to help the body lose water that is in excess in the tissues. Water loss facilitated by such a medication or substance takes place in the kidneys.

Ejaculate - A fluid that comes from the penis during intercourse. It is composed of fluids from the prostate and seminal vesicles and sperm cells from the testes.

Electrolyte - A chemical element necessary in our body for various reactions and processes. Sodium and potassium are very important ones.

Embolism - When blood clots that form in blood vessels, both veins and arteries, break loose, they are carried in the blood streams to different organs where they will cause damage, e.g., clots from the left side of the heart via an artery to the brain or clots from a major vein in a leg to the right side of the heart and then to the lungs.

Enzyme - A chemical substance made in the body with a specific task or purpose. Some enzymes play definite roles in digestion. Others in cardiac or liver activity or in the changes made in cholesterol when converted to testosterone.

(Refer to the cholesterol diagram i.e. Desmolase, Hydroxylase, etc)

Gonad - Organs in the reproductive system. i.e. ovaries or testes

Gonadotropin - A hormone from the pituitary directed to another endocrine gland. i.e. Follicle stimulating hormone influencing the testes to produce testosterone.

Heart Attack - This is a general term for a serious interference with normal heart function. It has come to mean a change in arterial (coronary) blood flow to the heart musculature through blockade of the blood either partial or complete. It could mean however change in cardiac rhythm (arrhythmia) or problem with a damaged valve or even congestive heart failure. It is often called a cardiac accident as well.

Hypogonadal - An underactivity of a gonad. i.e. testes not producing enough testosterone

Injection - Placement of a substance usually a drug directly into a muscle or other ogran, but it could be fluids into a blood vessel either a vein or artery. Various terms that are associated are: intramuscular (Im), subcutaneous (Sub Q)-beneath the skin, intravenous (Iv)-into a vein.

Lipid Profile - A test for some or all the known components of the blood that have to do with lipid or fat-like substances circulating in the blood. i.e. Cholesterol, LDL, HDL, triglycerides and other substances

Regimen - A protocol, a plan of therapy, a set of steps for medical treatment

Steroid - A substance that has a specific chemical configuration or nucleus. These are all steroids. (Refer to the cholesterol conversion chart, page 11)

CONCLUSION

Medical care is costly — too costly at times, I believe. Nonetheless, overall careful evaluation on a periodic basis, of one's health and the effect of a hormonal regimen must be carried out by a capable, knowledgeable, and interested physician. This will insure a comfortable life with good health and safe progress in the masculinization process.

Hence, do not fail to continue with an appropriate plan for periodic medical evaluation.

It must be a cooperative effort. Each individual is in all reality "meddling" with their own genetic, biochemical and physical makeup. The individual should always follow directions and keep in contact with the physician as requested or required.

I hope the information given to you has been of help and that it can be an aid in making your approach to this therapy a lot less mysterious and a great deal more comfortable.